SKIN DEEP

A DERMATOLOGIST'S GUIDE TO THE SCIENCE OF SKIN CARE

NANCY LEE SILVERBERG, MD

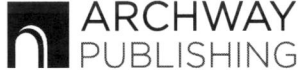

Copyright © 2023 Nancy Lee Silverberg, MD.

All rights reserved. No part of this book may be used or reproduced by any means, graphic, electronic, or mechanical, including photocopying, recording, taping or by any information storage retrieval system without the written permission of the author except in the case of brief quotations embodied in critical articles and reviews.

Archway Publishing books may be ordered through booksellers or by contacting:

Archway Publishing
1663 Liberty Drive
Bloomington, IN 47403
www.archwaypublishing.com
844-669-3957

Because of the dynamic nature of the Internet, any web addresses or links contained in this book may have changed since publication and may no longer be valid. The views expressed in this work are solely those of the author and do not necessarily reflect the views of the publisher, and the publisher hereby disclaims any responsibility for them.

Any people depicted in stock imagery provided by Getty Images are models, and such images are being used for illustrative purposes only. Certain stock imagery © Getty Images.

ISBN: 978-1-6657-2636-8 (sc)
ISBN: 978-1-6657-2637-5 (e)

Library of Congress Control Number: 2022912332

Print information available on the last page.

Archway Publishing rev. date: 05/04/2023

ACKNOWLEDGEMENTS

My biggest thank you goes to my husband, Dr. Larry Silverberg, for his never-ending love and unwavering support of all I do. This book would not have been possible without him.

I would also like to thank Platinum/West Dermatology and my staff, especially Linda Vertheim, Amber Lachmund and Stephanie Murphy, for their support and encouragement during the writing of this book. A special thank you goes to Carrie Lande, who plodded through the first draft of my manuscript and made wonderful and helpful suggestions.

Finally, thanks to the editors and the team at Archway publishing who helped shape this book and bring it to life.

CONTENTS

Acknowledgements..v
Foreword..ix

Chapter 1 1
  The Sea of Products:
  Snake Oil Versus Reality

Chapter 2 9
  Aging:
  Can I Stay Young Forever?

Chapter 3 15
  Sunscreens:
  Is There Really a Healthy Tan?

Chapter 4 25
  Moisturizers:
  The Slippery Slope

Chapter 5 35
  Alpha Hydroxy Acids:
  The Other Fruits

Chapter 6 39
  Vitamin A Derivatives:
  Retinoids and Friends

Chapter 7 47
  Peptides:
  Friends of Collagen

Chapter 8 51
Antioxidants:
Free Radicals Beware!

Chapter 9 57
Growth Factors:
Factors, Not Hormones

Chapter 10 65
Cleansers:
The Good, the Bad, and the Irritating

Chapter 11 71
Hair Products:
Shining, Gleaming, Streaming

Chapter 12 83
Nail Products:
Tools, Not Jewels

Chapter 13 91
Acne Products:
I'm Too Old For This!

Chapter 14 103
Preservatives:
To Preserve or Not to Preserve

Chapter 15 107
Conclusion

References 109

FOREWORD

I am a board-certified dermatologist who has been in practice in Newport Beach, California for thirty-six years. I spent my professional life listening to patients complain about the confusing array of skin care products and the advertising claims barraging them. It all left them wondering what was worth spending their money on. My goal in this book is to clarify, in a straightforward and simple manner, which products and ingredients are supported by scientific data, and to help consumers navigate the maze of skin care products available over the counter in retail stores and online.

I hope that this book will help you in the same way that I was able to educate my patients.

CHAPTER 1

The Sea of Products: Snake Oil Versus Reality

When you walk down the skin care aisle of a drug or department store, you are probably overwhelmed by the sheer number of products, all with appealing names and fancy packaging. The products often make dramatic and outlandish claims that they can reverse aging, diminish fine lines and wrinkles, reduce puffiness and dark circles, and promise "younger looking skin without drastic measures."

If these claims seem too good to be true, you are partially correct. In one study, as many as 82 percent of cosmetic product claims were found to be, at the very least, misleading or, at most, outright lies (Fowler et al., 2015)

The skin care market is predicted to reach $185 billion by 2025 (Wood, 2020). So is it any wonder that the largest square footage in department and drug stores is devoted to this industry? Is it surprising that a majority of these claims are downright deceptive?

How is this possible? Moreover, how is this legal?

This is possible because according to the Federal Food, Drug, and Cosmetics Act, a cosmetic product is anything intended to be rubbed, poured, sprinkled, sprayed, introduced into, or otherwise applied to the human body for the purpose of cleansing, beautifying, promoting attractiveness, or altering appearance.

A drug, on the other hand, is a product that is intended to affect the structure or function of the body of humans or other animals. Drugs must undergo strict testing to prove that their claims of affecting the structure or function of an organ (such as the skin) are true, and that the product is safe.

It is no surprise, then, that most companies avoid the testing process altogether and simply market their products as cosmetics, saying that they are intended to beautify the skin. They skirt around actual claims of altering the structure or function of the skin, and simply state that their product makes it more beautiful, supple, or smooth. The meaningless claim "dermatologist tested" simply indicates that one dermatologist somewhere tried it, regardless of whether he or she liked it.

In policing health and fitness claims, the Federal Trade Commission (FTC), the government watchdog agency for truth in advertising and partner to the Food and Drug Administration (FDA), has largely ignored the cosmetics industry. The FTC chooses to focus instead on the overwhelming number of fraudulent and sometimes dangerous weight loss foods and dietary supplements.

So how can the savvy consumer know which claims are true, and therefore, which products are worth purchasing? There is actual data from clinical trials that is published in peer-reviewed medical and scientific journals. In the following chapters, I will share my knowledge, as a skin specialist/dermatologist, about this data with you, the consumer.

That is the impetus for this book. My goal is to let you know, in the simplest way possible, which products (specifically, which ingredients) are backed by data and science and which are not. This book is not meant to be exhaustive, and if it were, I think you might end up feeling more confused about skin products than before you read it (or after you fell asleep!).

I am simply going to tell you about ingredients that, backed by scientific data, do what they say they do. I am not promoting or selling any specific product, and if I mention the name of a particular one, it is only as an example of something that may contain an effective ingredient.

To have a better understanding of how and why products work or do not work, we will first look at the structure of the skin.

Skin Structure

The skin, the largest organ of the human body and its primary protection, covers the body's entire external surface and serves as a physical barrier against the environment. It has many functions, including protection against ultraviolet (UV) light, trauma, pathogens, microorganisms, and toxins. The skin also plays a role in immunologic surveillance, sensory perception, control of water loss, and general homeostasis.

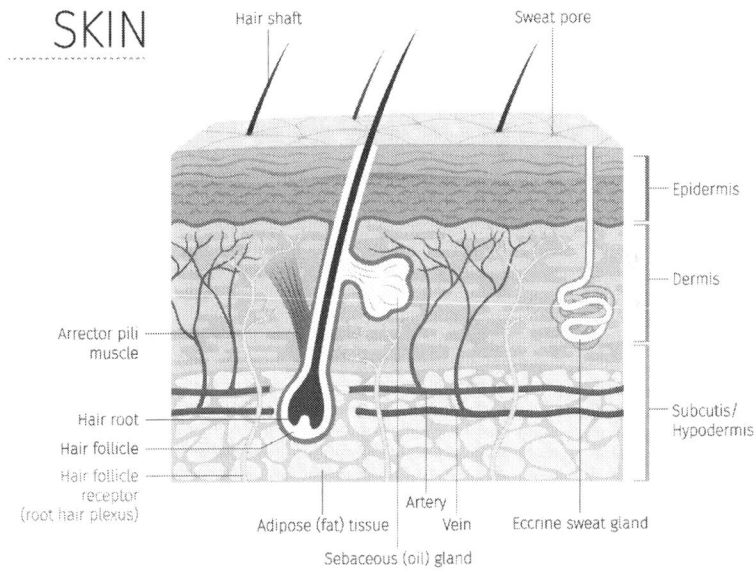

Not surprisingly, the skin has a complex architecture that can vary depending on body location. It consists of three layers. Starting from the surface, they are the epidermis, the dermis, and the subcutaneous tissue, or subcutis. Each has its own specific cells and respective functions. Skin appendages, such as hair follicles, sebaceous glands, and sweat glands, also play various roles in its overall function.

Epidermis

The epidermis forms a protective barrier against environmental influences. The external layer of the epidermis, the stratum corneum, is made up of dead cells (corneocytes) embedded in epidermal fats (lipids). The cells in the epidermis gradually migrate from the lower level (the basal layer) up to the outer layer and are continually shed. These dead cells are the flakes that you see on the surface of your skin.

The epidermal lipids and corneocytes resemble a brick wall. The corneocytes are thought of as the bricks, and the layers of lipids, found between the cells, are the mortar. The lipid mortar is the main barrier for water passing through the external layer of the epidermis (stratum corneum).

Dermis

The dermis is immediately below the epidermis and consists of dense connective tissue, composed of collagen and elastin fibers. Collagen gives skin its substance and fullness. The elastin fibers provide its snap-back quality. In addition, hair follicles, sweat glands, oil glands, and blood vessels are present in the dermis.

Subcutis

The subcutis, or subcutaneous tissue, is composed mostly of fat cells; it cushions the body and protects it from trauma.

In the next chapters, I will explain how the various ingredients of products interact with the skin and related hair and nails.

Aging: Can I Stay Young Forever?

CHAPTER 2

Aging is a natural part of life. Humans are born, go through a period of growth and development, reach maturity, gradually go through senescence, or aging, and die. Life is maturation.

The goal of antiaging is not about removing the process of aging, or even about necessarily prolonging life. Dying young is, of course, the only way to completely avoid aging, and for most of us, that is not a desirable option.

Patients ask me every day for antiaging therapy. If we were to take that request to the extreme, would they want to look like a child or even a teenager? When I ask them that question, the answer is overwhelmingly negative. Their answer is remarkably consistent: "I want to look as good as I can for my age."

I encourage patients to embrace the inevitable aging process. The goal is to look as good and be as healthy as one can be for a given age. As

Dr. Barbara Gilchrest has said, "Looking and feeling wonderful at a mature age is antiaging" (Gilchrest, 1989).

Skin Aging and Photoaging

Aging of the skin is broadly divided into two categories: intrinsic aging and photoaging. Intrinsic aging is chronologic aging; it is related to the passage of time. Photoaging is aging that occurs as a result of ultraviolet exposure, both from sunlight and from artificial sources, such as tanning beds.

Human skin, like all other organs, ages over time. Intrinsic aging of the skin is seen in sun-protected areas of the body and is characterized by thinning of the skin, loss of elasticity, increased fragility, fine wrinkling, and decreased wound healing. Because older skin is thinner, the skin appears translucent and blood vessels are more visible. Skin cells from older people, which are cultured and grown in the laboratory, have decreased life spans and a diminished response to growth factors when compared to skin cells from younger individuals (Gilchrest, 1996).

Photoaging is the term used to describe changes in chronically sun-exposed skin. Photoaged skin is characterized by fine and coarse wrinkles, laxity, roughness, mottled pigmentation, leathery texture, dryness, and yellowed coloring. Most of these changes are caused by multiple, brief exposures to ultraviolet light sources, not necessarily intended to produce tanning (Drake, 1996). Most of the skin signs we associate with aging are due to sun exposure.

Chronologic (or intrinsic) aging, the aging which occurs in non-sun-exposed areas, shows thinning of all layers of the skin, decreased oil production, and decreased growth of body hair. We can look at areas on our bodies (such as the buttocks) that have had little to no exposure to sun and compare them to areas that were chronically exposed. We see that the exposed skin and the non-exposed skin often look like they come from two completely different individuals.

The epidermis, or the outer layer of the skin, is constantly turning over and being shed (these are the dead cells you see as flaky skin). The rate of this turnover continually slows down by as much as 50 percent from age twenty to age seventy (Cerimele, 1970). The dermis, or the deeper layer of the skin, becomes thinner and more fragile due to a decrease in collagen, elastin fibers, and proteins.

There is also a decrease in the number of blood vessels and oil glands in the skin with age. All of these changes result in thin, fragile, and saggy skin with a yellowish appearance. Minor trauma can result in bruising or breaking of the skin, and wounds heal more slowly.

The picture below is a split image of facial skin in which one side has been protected from environmental assaults and the other side has been repeatedly exposed to the environment, especially ultraviolet light. The exposed skin shows fine and coarse wrinkling, mottled pigmentation, laxity and leathery texture compared to the protected side, which has minimal changes.

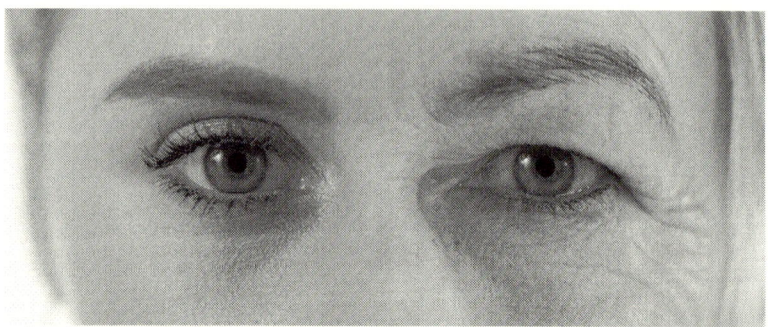

Comparing a sun-exposed area, like the face or arm, to a non-sun-exposed area, like the buttocks, is a perfect example of the difference between photoaging and intrinsic aging. The two areas of this patient's skin were composed of the same DNA, lived in the same location, had the same diet, drank the same water, and were exposed to the same environmental factors—with the one exception of exposure to ultraviolet light.

So, are any of these changes preventable or reversible? We will look at what is available and what is possible.

Sunscreens: Is There Really a Healthy Tan?

CHAPTER 3

Ultraviolet radiation reaching the earth's surface contains about 5 percent ultraviolet B (short wave, or sunburn, rays) and 95 percent ultraviolet A (long wave or black light). Ultraviolet B (UVB for short) affects the more superficial layers of the skin, causing sunburn and ultimately skin darkening, or tanning. Ultraviolet A (UVA) penetrates more deeply into the skin; it leads to darkening of the skin and, occasionally, redness. UVA is the main type of light used in tanning beds, and has been erroneously promoted as the safe way to tan. Unlike UVB rays, UVA is not absorbed by the ozone layer, which means that there is less of a natural barrier to UVA rays.

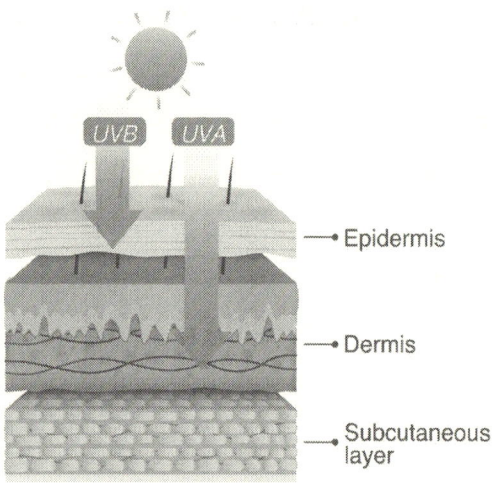

Both types of ultraviolet light cause the changes in the skin we refer to as photoaging—thinning, loss of elasticity, mottling, and wrinkles. They can also damage the skin's cellular DNA, creating genetic mutations that can lead to all types of skin cancer. Interestingly, even though UVA has lower energy levels than UVB, due to its deeper penetration into the skin, it seems to contribute more than UVB to premature aging and skin cancers. In addition, the largest amount of ultraviolet radiation coming from the sun is UVA.

New research from the American Academy of Dermatology found that rates of melanoma—the most lethal form of skin cancer—have increased by nearly 800 percent among women between the ages of eighteen and thirty-nine since 1970 (Guy, 2015). Other less lethal and more common forms of skin cancer (basal cell carcinoma and squamous cell carcinoma) have also increased dramatically. While we do not know all of the reasons behind this frightening rise in skin cancer rates—which may be due to better education and diagnosis, more revealing clothing styles, and other factors—we do know that the primary cause is exposure to UV radiation from the sun. We also know ways to prevent it.

While ultraviolet light exposure is most damaging to fair-skinned Caucasians with light hair and/or light eyes, it is also damaging to darker skinned individuals. While darker skinned races tend to sunburn less readily and tan more easily, the damage from ultraviolet light can still be significant, and protective measures are equally important for them as well.

There are simple ways to minimize UV exposure, such as avoidance of the sun between the most intense hours of 10:00 a.m. and 2:00 p.m., wearing sun protective clothing, UPF (Ultraviolet Protection

Factor) fabric hats, and sunglasses. There are also, of course, a wide variety of sunscreen products available to everyone.

Sunscreens

Sunscreens are available as organic sunscreens (also referred to as chemical) and inorganic sunscreens (also referred to as chemical free). This is really a meaningless distinction, since a chemical by definition is any substance consisting of matter; referring to an inorganic, typically mineral-based, sunscreen as chemical free is a misnomer.

The common rating system of sunscreens is the SPF, which stands for Sun Protection Factor. We are all familiar with these numbers, but what do they actually mean? The SPF is a measure of the effectiveness of a sunscreen formulation. This factor is determined by assessing individual sensitivity to sunburn with and without the sunscreen.

SPF=time of sun exposure to produce redness *without* sunscreen versus time of sun exposure to produce redness *with* sunscreen

SPF is defined as the amount of solar radiation

required to produce redness in sunscreen-protected skin divided by the amount required to produce redness in non-sunscreen protected skin. For instance, a sunscreen with an SPF of 15 will prevent your skin from getting red for approximately fifteen times longer than usual. If you start to burn in ten minutes, sunscreen with SPF 15 will prevent burning for about 150 minutes, or 2.5 hours.

The American Academy of Dermatology recommends using sunscreen with an SPF between 15 and 50 (SPF ratings higher than 50 have not been proven more effective than SPF 50). A sunscreen with an SPF of 15 protects against about 93 percent of UVB rays, and one with an SPF of 30 protects against 97 percent of UVB rays.

Remember, UVA comprises 95 percent of the radiation reaching us and it is not absorbed by the ozone layer, as UVB is; the SPF ratings on sunscreen labels *only* apply to UVB. All the hype about SPF and the numbers game—Is 15 enough? Is 50 too much?—*only* applies to that 5 percent of radiation that is UVB. There is *no* reference or numerical system that tells us how much protection we get from UVA—the most dangerous source of ultraviolet rays. The FDA will likely come up with a numerical system to assess the effectiveness of sunscreens against UVA in the future, but as of now, we have to pay attention to the products' ingredients to assure that we get adequate protection from UVA radiation.

One last note: it is important to be generous when applying sunscreen, and to make sure to cover all exposed skin surfaces, including the neck and behind the ears. A rule of thumb is to use a shot glass worth of sunscreen per application on the body.

Let us look at the two classifications of sunscreens, inorganic and organic, often referred to (inaccurately) as chemical-free and chemical.

Inorganic sunscreens typically include minerals such as zinc oxide or titanium dioxide, which act as physical sunblocks. They reflect a broad range of ultraviolet rays in both the UVA and UVB spectrum, similar to how white paint reflects light. The white-colored noses on beachgoers in the 1960s and 1970s were due to these compounds, and most people found them cosmetically unacceptable for daily use. Because manufacturers now make the inorganic particles much smaller (micronized), they have a much more transparent appearance and smoother application than the toothpaste-like consistency and color of the old zinc and titanium preparations.

Organic sunscreens work by absorbing ultraviolet radiation through their bonds, like a sponge. As the bonds absorb UV radiation, the components of the sunscreen slowly break down. Organic sunscreens almost exclusively absorb ultraviolet in the short-wave range, or ultraviolet B. Common organic ingredients are avobenzone, aminobenzoic acid, octyl salicylate, octocrylene, and oxybenzone.

Some of the chemicals in sunscreens (specifically oxybenzone) have recently come under fire for possibly being carcinogenic or otherwise harmful (Suh et al, 2020). Studies have found that oxybenzone can be absorbed through the skin and may act as a hormone disrupter, possibly interfering with the body's natural hormone production. Studies have been cited that involve feeding large amounts of oxybenzone to rats. It would take an individual 277 years of sunscreen use to achieve the equivalent systemic dose that produced effects in these rat studies. There has been no conclusive evidence that oxybenzone is harmful to humans (Wang, Burnett, and Lim 2011). However, some researchers have suggested not using sunscreens containing this chemical on children or pregnant women. In addition, research has also suggested that some organic chemical sunscreen ingredients can have toxic impacts on a variety of aquatic organisms, including corals and marine life. The FDA is committed to doing further research on these products.

Vitamin D and Sunscreen

Vitamin D is critical for humans—it helps keep bones strong by regulating calcium levels and helps to prevent osteoporosis. It is also important to the immune system and may play a role in preventing cancer and other diseases. The skin manufactures vitamin D when it is exposed to sunlight. Ultraviolet B interacts with a precursor protein in the skin to convert that precursor into vitamin D3, the active form of vitamin D.

So what happens when we use sunscreen and

other sun protective measures? Is there a minimum amount of unprotected sun exposure that people should have to ensure they do not develop vitamin D deficiency?

Numerous clinical studies have shown that daily sunscreen use rarely causes vitamin D deficiency (Neale et al, 2019). It takes such a small amount of UVB exposure to produce vitamin D, and sun protection is rarely thorough enough to prevent that amount. However, individuals who apply sunscreen generously and religiously wear hats and UV-protective clothing do have a slightly higher risk of developing vitamin D insufficiency. It is easy to obtain enough vitamin D (600 IU) from a combination of diet and supplements. Vitamin D levels can easily be checked with a blood test, and if it is below the recommended level of 30 ng/mL, you can replace it with supplements.

In summary, the evidence is overwhelming for the many benefits of sun protection. The Skin Cancer Foundation recommends daily use of an SPF of 15 or over, broad-spectrum (UVA-UVB) sunscreen. This is in addition to other forms of sun protection, such as avoiding the peak sunlight hours between 10 and 2, sun-protective clothing, hats, and UV filtering sunglasses. Both the U.S. Department of Health and Human Services and the World Health Organization have identified ultraviolet light as a proven human carcinogen, with studies linking it to about 90 percent of nonmelanoma skin cancers (basal cell carcinoma and squamous cell carcinoma) and about 85 percent of melanomas, as well as premature skin aging (Watts, 2018). In addition, UV radiation harms the eyes and can cause cataracts, eyelid cancers, and other ocular skin cancers, including melanomas.

Protection from the sun's ultraviolet rays is important on a daily basis, not just when you're planning to be outside. Healthy skin is protected skin—there is no such thing as a healthy tan.

Shun the sun!

CHAPTER 4

Moisturizers: The Slippery Slope

There is no consensus regarding the definition of a moisturizer. The term moisturizer is a marketing term with little or no scientific meaning. It was coined by Madison Avenue marketers to describe various creams and lotions. However, since everyone knows what we're talking about when we use the word moisturizer, I will continue to use that term here.

The main function of this group of products called moisturizers is to remedy dry skin. Dryness is a result of decreased water content of the stratum corneum, the outer layer of skin. For skin to look and feel normal, the water content of this layer must be above 10 percent. Water is lost through evaporation to the environment and must be replenished by water from the lower epidermal and dermal layers. The job of the stratum corneum is to maintain this moisture so that the skin won't feel rough, scaly, and dry.

Skin typically is dryer in less humid environments, which cause more epidermal water loss, and in older skin, where the stratum corneum lacks the ability to hold in water effectively.

Ingredients

Most moisturizers are comprised of formulations that are either oil-in-water (water is the dominant phase) or water-in-oil (oil is the dominant phase). Whether these formulations, known as emulsions, are considered creams or lotions depends on their relative percentage of water—those with higher water concentrations that are more pourable are generally considered lotions. Nevertheless, if you look at the ingredient list, you'll notice that water is usually the first ingredient in most creams and lotions. When you apply the product to the skin, some of the water evaporates, but some soaks into the top layer (the stratum corneum). To avoid immediate evaporation from the skin surface, an oily substance is mixed, or emulsified, with the water. Ointments, which are emulsions with mostly oil (at least 80 percent), tend to feel greasier and are glossier in appearance.

There are three main classes of moisturizers depending on their function: emollients, humectants, and occlusives.

Emollients do not actually moisturize skin, but they cause a slippery or smooth feeling on the skin. Skin slip plays a major role in consumer satisfaction. Common emollients are fatty acids, lipids, fatty alcohols, ceramides, cholesterol, and vegetable waxes. Virtually all moisturizers contain emollients in some form.

Humectants pull water into the stratum corneum both from the environment and from deeper layers of the skin. However, when the humidity is low, there is so little water in the air that almost all of the water comes from the inside out. Common humectants are glycerin, propylene glycol, urea, hyaluronic acid, and some proteins. Humectants are usually paired with occlusive ingredients that trap the moisture the humectants draw into the stratum corneum.

Occlusives form an inert layer on the skin and physically block the evaporation of water from the stratum corneum. Most occlusives contain petrolatum, mineral oils (derived from petrolatum), lanolin, liquid paraffin, and silicones.

Location, Location, Location

Moisturizers and other skin care products do not know the difference between your face, neck, eyes, body, hands, or feet. They do not know the difference between night and day. Yet the marketing is so powerful for these location-specific products that most people wouldn't dream of using their foot cream on their face. The result? More products on the market and more money spent by consumers.

There are some minor differences (in type and number) between these products which are worth understanding so that you, the consumer, can make your best choice.

Face creams are generally made of oil-in-water emulsions for a thinner, nonglossy appearance. They are designed to be non-greasy and non-acne forming with an emphasis on aesthetic appearance. For oily skin, silicone is often used for its slippery feel, and kaolin and talc are often added for their oil absorbency.

Eye creams are formulated like any other facial moisturizer, and it is a myth that a separate cream is necessary for the eye area. Sometimes some of the more irritating ingredients are removed, like fragrance, exotic oils, or vitamins. The skin of the eye area is no different from the skin on the cheekbone. If a facial moisturizer isn't formulated safely enough to be applied around the eye, then it surely shouldn't be applied to the cheekbone, an inch or two away.

Hand, Foot, and Body Creams tend to have higher oil content and come in a variety of preparations including cream, lotion, mousse, and ointment. There is no difference between the products used for the hands, feet, and body. Because the hands and feet are subject to more severe dryness, these products are more commonly found in cream and ointment formulations. Body lotions often have a thinner consistency, especially if they're going to be applied to hairy areas.

Female patients may prefer a product with a rich texture; however, a rich texture does not necessarily imply a better moisturizer. Richness can be created with water-soluble gums that impart a silky feel but do not create better moisture retention.

Oily and Acne-Prone Skin

Most cosmetic companies clearly label which products are designed for oily, normal and dry skin. Comedogenesis (the tendency to produce blackheads in a rabbit ear model) or acnegenesis (the tendency to produce acne lesions in human skin) are studied in skin preparations and used to label a product's ability to induce acne lesions. Non-comedogenic or non-acnegenic should be clearly marked on a product intended for acne-prone skin.

Oil-free labelling can be confusing. Oil-free products typically contain water and propylene glycol (a slip agent) but do not contain mineral oil, other lipids, or petrolatum. However, numerous slip agents that can still predispose skin to acne can be added to a product labelled oil-free. It is important for the product to contain the label of non-comedogenic or non-acnegenic in addition to oil-free. (See more information about acne products in Chapter 13.)

Other Ingredients

There are numerous other ingredients added to moisturizers to enhance their benefit and appeal to consumers.

- A frequent additive to skin products is Aloe *(Aloe barbadensis),* of which more than 300 species are available. Evidence to support its role as a moisturizer is lacking, although its role in healing burns and minor wounds due to its anti-inflammatory, antibacterial, vasodilator action has been shown.
- Oatmeal *(Avena sativa)* for soothing irritated skin has been well known for decades.
- Proteins or simple amino acids (the breakdown products of protein) such as collagen, elastin, and keratin are popular additives to moisturizers. These molecules are generally too large to penetrate the skin barrier, but may function as humectants by holding water on the skin surface.

- Vitamins are also common additives to face creams, though their penetration through the skin is doubtful, and their usefulness in moisturizing skin is unproven. Like proteins, they may have some function as humectants.
- Fragrances and coloring agents are present in skin care products more for their cosmetic enhancement than for any true role in moisturization. The color or odor of plain moisturizers can often be unappealing, and cosmetic companies have found that sales often increase dramatically with these additives. Unfortunately, they can be sensitizing and cause dermatitis in sensitive individuals.
- Preservatives are added to all products to inhibit the growth of bacteria and fungi. They are essential to any product other than single-use products (like certain eye products). Phenoxyethanol and parabens are the most frequently used products in moisturizers, although they can cause sensitivity and there has been debate about their safety (addressed later in this book in Chapter 14).

- Emulsifying agents are added to prevent the natural tendency of oil and water to separate. Most emulsifying agents are detergents, most commonly laureth 4 and 9, ethylene glycol, octoxinols, and nonoxinols.
- Liposomes are a newer technology that uses minute spherical sacs of phospholipid molecules enclosing a water droplet to deliver products into the epidermis.

In summary, moisturizers make skin look and feel smoother and softer, and can also help makeup go on better. Do they prevent wrinkles or reverse aging? Despite the alluring marketing and extravagant claims made by manufacturers, the answer is a simple no. Let us look at products that may actually affect the skin.

Alpha Hydroxy Acids: The Other Fruits

CHAPTER 5

Alpha hydroxy acids (AHAs) are a group of natural acids found in plants. AHAs include glycolic acid (found in sugar cane), citric acid (found in citrus fruits), lactic acid (found in sour milk), malic acid (found in apples), and tartaric acid (found in grapes). AHAs are water soluble, which means they dissolve in water.

Glycolic acid is the most well-known and commonly used AHA for its well-documented anti-aging benefit (Ditre, 1996) and ability to improve hyperpigmentation and acne-prone skin.

How do alpha hydroxy acids work? They remove the top layers of the stratum corneum (the dead skin cells on the outer surface of the epidermis) and promote cell turnover. Microscopically, they have been shown to increase epidermal thickness, decrease abnormality of epidermal cells and cause even dispersion of pigment cells. In the dermis (the middle skin layer), the AHAs stimulate collagen fiber synthesis and cause elastic fibers to be longer, thicker, and more abundant.

In terms of visible results, these products cause thickening of the skin (reversing some of the tissue paper like thinness we see in older skin), more elasticity (that snap-back quality we see in young skin), and more even pigmentation (reducing the appearance of age spots). AHAs can also help treat and prevent recurring acne.

Minor side effects can occur with these products, especially when beginning treatment. These include burning, itching, dermatitis, and even occasional blisters. Because they remove the top layer of skin cells, they can also make skin more sensitive to the sun's ultraviolet light (UVA and UVB rays). Most of these side effects are temporary, and diminish after continued use.

The AHAs are not the only hydroxy acids on the market. Beta hydroxy acid (BHA), most commonly in the form of salicylic acid, is closely related chemically to the AHAs (with only one additional carbon atom). Because the BHAs are oil soluble, in contrast to AHAs which are water soluble, the BHAs are generally considered to be a better treatment for acne, since they are attracted to oil and can penetrate deeply into oily pores.

The BHAs can have many of the same temporary side effects as the AHAs, such as irritation and sun sensitivity, although these are typically less severe in the BHAs.

Newer agents, the polyhydroxy acids (PHAs) are considered cousins of alpha hydroxy acids; they are, in fact, second-generation AHAs. The most common PHAs are gluconolactone, galactose, and lactobionic acid. Similar to the AHAs, PHAs work by exfoliating dead skin cells on the surface, resulting in a more even skin tone and texture. However, the molecules of PHAs are much larger and therefore cannot penetrate as deeply as AHAs and BHAs. They work exclusively on the surface of the skin, and because of this, are much less irritating than their AHA and BHA counterparts. These may be a better choice for people with sensitive skin.

All of the hydroxy acids, when used in higher concentrations, can be applied to the skin as a chemical peel. Because they weaken the connections between the cells in the top layer of the skin, they remove more of the dead skin cells, giving the skin a refreshed and glowing look. They can also reduce the appearance of wrinkles, sunspots, and acne scars. These are available in lower concentrations, for at home peels, or higher concentrations for in-office peeling.

In summary, the evidence showing the effectiveness of the hydroxy acids is abundant and well-documented. AHAs, such as glycolic acid and lactic acid, penetrate the skin more deeply, and are best suited for normal to dry skin with aging changes. BHAs, such as salicylic acid, are better suited for oily, acne-prone skin, and are attracted to oily pores, dissolving sebum and dead skin cells. PHAs, such as gluconolactone, work for all skin types, but are ideal for people with sensitive or intolerant skin, due to their larger molecular size and more superficial penetration.

Finally, the hydroxy acids can be mixed together. Cocktails of two or even all three types of acids have been marketed to address fine lines, pigmentation, and aging skin, though these should be approached with caution. They can also be combined with humectants and other ingredients since they increase penetration of these products.

CHAPTER 6

Vitamin A Derivatives: Retinoids and Friends

Retinoids are a huge family of compounds derived from vitamin A. These compounds include both natural and synthetic derivatives. Retinoids are required for a vast number of biological processes, including reproduction, vision, growth, and cell growth and differentiation.

The most studied retinoid is tretinoin (also known as retinoic acid), which the FDA approved in 1971 for acne treatment under the brand name RetinA. After RetinA came into widespread use, it did not take long for more mature patients to notice an improvement in fine lines and wrinkles, age spots, and smoothness of the skin. Abundant, well-controlled medical studies have documented the impressive effects of tretinoin on photodamaged skin on both a microscopic and clinical level (Weiss et al, 1988, Kang and Voorhees, 1998).

What does tretinoin do to the skin, and how does it work?

Tretinoin induces the production of procollagen (the precursor to collagen) in the skin, and reduces the breakdown of collagen by inhibiting the natural enzymes that destroy collagen. The overall effect is a thickening of the dermal (or middle) layer of the skin, which reduces fine lines and wrinkles. I hear claims repeatedly made from non-medical personnel that tretinoin thins the skin and thus should be avoided in older people. Studies have repeatedly shown quite the opposite—it increases the thickness of the skin by as much as 33 percent (Bhawan, 1991). In addition, tretinoin stimulates the production of new blood vessels in the dermis, giving the skin a less sallow appearance, often described as a "rosy glow."

As discussed in Chapter 2, the skin cells in the epidermis, or the outer layer of the skin, are constantly turning over and being shed, and the rate of this transit gradually slows down with age. Regular use of tretinoin significantly speeds up this transit time of cells migrating from the lower level to the outer layer of the epidermis, bringing the transit time to rates much closer to the rates of younger skin. This gives skin a fresher, more youthful look, as opposed to the chalky, dull appearance of aged skin. It also reduces the clumping of melanin pigment, decreasing age spots and giving the skin a more evenly pigmented appearance.

Minor adverse effects of tretinoin are common, especially during the first three months of therapy. As many as 70 percent of patients experience redness, flaking, and mild burning during the first few weeks of use, and these adverse effects often lead them to discontinue using the product. After all, tretinoin is purported to improve the look of the skin—why continue when the skin looks red, irritated, and scaly?

It is important to recognize that during the first three months of therapy, side effects are prominent and beneficial therapeutic effects are minimal. With regular and continued use, side effects diminish and the beneficial effects become apparent. Beneficial effects of tretinoin do not become apparent until about twelve weeks of use, and these benefits continue to improve over six and even twelve months. The side effects of redness, flaking, and irritation gradually subside over that period of time, so it is critical to focus on the long-term benefits of this product and persevere through the initial weeks of therapy.

There are some tricks to minimize the side effects of tretinoin. Some practitioners recommend using it only every other day for the first few weeks, and then gradually working up to nightly applications. Tretinoin should also be applied to a bone-dry face; wait at least fifteen minutes after cleansing the face before applying it to lessen irritation caused by moisture on the skin. Retinoids increase the skin's sensitivity to sunlight, especially during the first weeks of therapy, so they should only be applied at nighttime, and sunscreen should always be worn during the day. After a few months of therapy, the skin's response to ultraviolet light seems to return to normal (but continued daily sunscreen use is still recommended).

Other Retinoids

Retinol, or all-trans retinol, is vitamin A alcohol, one of the natural retinoids. It is a precursor for the synthesis of retinoic acid (tretinoin). Although retinol has been used in over-the-counter cosmetic products since 1984, it wasn't until 1995 that it was shown that application of retinol on normal human skin induces epidermal thickening and stimulates collagen synthesis (Kang, 1995). However, it was observed that retinol is twenty times less potent than tretinoin, and that it requires conversion to retinoic acid (in the skin) to become active. In addition, retinol is extremely unstable and easily degrades to biologically inactive forms when exposed to light and air. Interestingly, retinol showed only minimal signs of skin reddening and irritation.

Clearly, retinol is an effective over-the-counter product for the treatment of aging skin. While it causes less irritancy than tretinoin, retinol is much less potent and less stable than tretinoin.

Retinol Derivatives

Retinol derivatives have been developed in order to improve the chemical stability of retinol. Retinol derivatives, like retinyl acetate, retinyl palmitate, and retinyl propionate, have been widely used in cosmetic products in place of retinol. While there have been some early studies in mice suggesting increased collagen formation and epidermal thickening, convincing double-blind studies in humans are still lacking.

Retinaldehyde

Retinaldehyde is a precursor to retinoic acid (tretinoin). Like retinol, it is available over-the-counter and does not require a prescription. It is formed as an intermediate product in the transformation of retinol to retinoic acid in human skin cells. It transforms into retinoic acid in the skin. Multiple, well-controlled studies have shown an increase in skin thickness and a decrease in visible wrinkling with retinaldehyde. It causes less irritation that tretinoin, but also has lower potency.

In conclusion, retinaldehyde is an over-the-counter retinoid useful in the treatment of photoaged skin, with a lower frequency of irritation than tretinoin.

Tazarotene

Tazarotene is a synthetic retinoid that was first approved for the treatment of psoriasis and acne in 1997. Subsequent clinical studies have shown tazarotene to cause a significant reduction in fine wrinkling, pigment mottling, and overall photodamage. This has been shown in double-blinded studies both in comparison to placebo (plain vehicle) and tretinoin cream. In some cases, its effect on photoaging has surpassed that of tretinoin (Kang et al, 2005).

Like all retinoids, tazarotene causes irritation (which may be more pronounced than tretinoin) during the first few weeks of use. It is available only by prescription.

Adapalene

Adapalene is considered to be a third-generation synthetic retinoid which was approved for the prescription-only treatment of acne in 1996. In 2016, the FDA approved adapalene for over-the-counter use. Because it has a very selective receptor uptake, it causes significantly less irritation than other retinoids.

So far, only one study has been carried out to assess the potential of adapalene in photoaging. This study, involving a small number of subjects, showed a significant improvement in wrinkles and other features of photoaging when compared to placebo (vehicle alone). Larger scale clinical trials must be carried out to validate these findings.

In summary, the family of retinoids are among the most promising agents available for the treatment of aging skin. Amongst the retinoids, tretinoin is the best-studied and most potent. Tretinoin, retinol, and retinaldehyde are naturally-occurring, and tazarotene and adapalene are synthetic. Tretinoin and tazarotene are the only two that require a doctor's prescription. All of the retinoids have the potential to cause irritation, although retinol, retinaldehyde, and adapalene are the least irritating and also the least potent.

CHAPTER 7

Peptides: Friends of Collagen

Peptides are molecules made up of short chains of amino acids. Peptides are the building blocks of proteins, of which the most important in the skin is collagen, the protein that gives skin its structure, firmness, and integrity. Some peptides occur naturally, often in plant sources, and some are synthetic. Many natural peptides are not stable in water solutions, which is a problem since the majority of skin care products contain water. Synthetic peptides are preferable in skin care because they are more stable in water and often more affordable.

There are numerous studies on the effects of peptides on skin aging, but most have involved very few subjects and are often not well controlled or published in scientific journals. However, this is an explosive topic in anti-aging skin care, and one that is worthy of notice and further study (Schagen, 2017).

Peptides can be divided into five classifications: signaling peptides, carrier peptides, neurotransmitter inhibitor peptides, enzyme inhibitor peptides, and structural peptides.

Signaling peptides are by far the most commonly used peptides in the cosmetic industry. Signaling peptides have different ways of increasing the proliferation of collagen, elastin, and glycosaminoglycans (substances that provide support to collagen and elastin). Procollagen segments (the precursors of collagen) can actually stimulate collagen production, but they can also signal skin cells that enough collagen has been broken down, so they can both help make more collagen or help the skin hold on to what it already has. Common signaling peptides have names like carnosine, and products ending in *peptide* or beginning in *palmitoyl*. They often have prefixes like di, tri, hexa, and oligo to describe how many amino acids make up the peptide.

Carrier peptides are probably the second most popular and well-examined skin care peptides. Carrier peptides hook up to another ingredient to facilitate their delivery to skin cells. The most common ingredient is copper, which is released in wounds to support healing. Copper can act as a signal and carrier peptide, promoting collagen, elastin, and glycosaminoglycan production as well as anti-inflammatory and antioxidant responses.

Neurotransmitter inhibitor peptides are less common than signaling and carrier peptides. These peptides appear to inhibit the release of acetylcholine, a neurotransmitter involved in muscle contractions. By decreasing the muscle contractions, they may cause the reduction and softening of wrinkles and fine lines.

Enzyme inhibitor peptides interfere with the activity of enzymes involved in a specific aging-related process. Specifically, they inhibit enzymes that mediate the breakdown of collagen and glycosaminoglycans. This results in the increase of these important proteins in the skin, decreasing wrinkling and thinning of the skin. The most common sources are soybeans, silk peptides, and rice proteins.

Structural keratin-based peptides are unique in that they specifically target dehydration and dryness in the skin, especially associated with soaps and cleansers. They are derived from keratin (the main constituent in hair and nails) and work by improving the integrity and water-holding capacity of the skin barrier. They are often combined with lipids to increase the emollient effect.

In conclusion, twenty years ago, no scientist ever thought that the topical use of natural or synthetic peptides for cosmetic use would be so effective. Since 2000, the use of peptides in skin care products has increased dramatically, and there is a significant amount of favorable scientific evidence.

Signaling peptides tell skin to make collagen and other dermal components. Carrier peptides increase the penetration of ingredients through the skin barrier. Neurotransmitter inhibitor peptides decrease muscular contractions in the skin. Enzyme inhibitor peptides decrease the enzymes that break down collagen. Structural peptides strengthen the skin's barrier. Peptides have been shown to increase the thickness of the skin, promote elasticity, and cause skin to appear smoother, firmer, and better hydrated.

Antioxidants: Free Radicals Beware!

CHAPTER 8

Antioxidants are a group of naturally occurring compounds that protect cells from damage.

To understand how antioxidants work, it is important to understand free radicals. Free radicals are unstable molecules that are missing an electron. These unstable molecules are created through cellular respiration, metabolic processes, and external stresses (like sunlight, pollution, radiation, and cigarette smoke). These highly reactive free radicals steal electrons from other molecules that are fundamental to normal homeostasis, such as proteins, lipids, or DNA. This creates inflammation and results in premature aging of the body, including the skin, as well as causing some types of skin cancers. Antioxidants work by donating an electron to the free radicals, which neutralizes them and prevents them from damaging cells and tissues. This is how antioxidants give a protective effect against aging and disease.

However, not all free radicals are bad. Some situations causing mild stress, like calorie restriction and physical activity, can generate free radicals. These free radicals can provoke an adaptive response, giving the body resistance to stress and infection and modulating the aging process. The problem occurs when there are too many free radicals compared to antioxidants, and the excess free radicals are available to damage cells.

Antioxidants aren't just one ingredient, so that word won't be listed on the product's ingredients list. There are a large number of antioxidants that all have one property in common: they fight free radicals, and help with the skin's natural regeneration process. Below is a list of some of the best-studied antioxidants.

Vitamin C, or L-ascorbic acid, is one of the most commonly used and widely studied antioxidants. Vitamin C is a powerful antioxidant that binds and removes free radicals from the skin, like those produced by exposure to ultraviolet light and pollutants. Therefore, it has a protective effect when applied to the skin before exposure to these elements. It also helps to stimulate collagen production and can help to fade dark spots. Vitamin C is quite unstable, and actually breaks down when exposed to light or air. Therefore, packaging is important—it must be in dark, airtight containers.

Vitamin E, or tocopherol, has been shown in animal models and human studies to combat sun damage. Scientific studies have demonstrated that vitamin E treatment can reduce UV-induced photodamage, decrease the risk of skin cancers, and stabilize the skin barrier (Addor, 2017). In addition to its antioxidant properties, vitamin E may also protect the skin by absorbing UV light, but since it is rapidly depleted by the UV light, it is often used in combination with other antioxidants. Specifically, vitamin C has been shown to stabilize and help regenerate vitamin E, making the combination of the two vitamins especially effective in fighting UV damage.

Ferulic acid is a plant-based antioxidant that fights free radicals and can boost the effectiveness of other antioxidants. Vitamin C is notoriously unstable, and ferulic acid is thought to help stabilize vitamin C while also increasing its photoprotection.

Vitamin B3, or niacinamide, is a powerful antioxidant found in many foods we eat, mostly meat. Studies have shown that topical application of vitamin B3 has many potential skin benefits, including increased skin hydration, reduced fine lines and wrinkles, minimized redness and blotchiness, and decreased pigmented spots. It can also help regulate the amount of oil the sebaceous glands produce, controlling sebum production in oily skin.

Green tea polyphenols, also known as catechins, have multiple antioxidant effects, including anti-inflammatory and anti-carcinogenic properties, and decreased collagen breakdown. Because of their powerful anti-inflammatory properties, the polyphenols help reduce redness, and they are especially good for sensitive skin.

Resveratrol is naturally found in berries, peanuts, red grapes, and--you guessed it--red wine. Resveratrol possesses antioxidant and anti-inflammatory properties. Scientific studies suggest that topically applied resveratrol protects against ultraviolet-induced photodamage, pigmentation, and collagen degradation. In other words, it may help brighten skin and reduce fine lines.

Curcumin is a polyphenol found in turmeric root, that bold, yellow-colored spice that is popular in Mediterranean foods. Curcumin decreases inflammation, fights free radicals, helps to fight oily skin and acne, and is photo-protective and anti-bacterial.

In summary, antioxidants are a diverse group of compounds that help protect the skin and prevent damage resulting from many environmental assaults, such as sunlight, pollution, radiation, and more. Because of their preventative function, they should be applied in the morning, before a moisturizer and sunscreen. Many antioxidants are fragile and not shelf-stable, so they must be packaged appropriately (and not left open to air). They are often combined with other antioxidants to increase stability.

Growth Factors: Factors, Not Hormones

CHAPTER 9

Growth factors were first discovered by two scientists in the 1950s, an achievement that earned them the Nobel Prize in Medicine in 1986. It was known at that time that a human begins as a single cell, which divides and then differentiates into many unique, specialized cells which form organs. These scientists showed that growth factors are responsible for regulating the cell's growth and differentiation.

Growth factors are found in abundance throughout the human body, and are produced by all types of cells. They communicate to receptors on other cells, and regulate cell replication, function, and differentiation. They regulate many cellular processes, like development, metabolism, and immune responses. In the skin, that may result in increased collagen and elastin formation, decreased inflammation, and improved wound healing. Growth factors have been compared to keys, and their receptors to locks: When the key clicks into the lock, it activates the cell to do things, like grow and divide, make more collagen and elastin, or increase blood flow. However, with age, that lock-and-key mechanism begins to get rusty, and the skin starts producing fewer growth factors, resulting in decreased amounts of collagen, elastin, and blood vessels. This results in aging, thin skin with loss of elasticity, and sallowness.

Growth factors can either be human-derived or synthetically produced, often from plant sources. Human growth factors usually come from human stem cells, often from many different sources. The fascinating property of stem cells—whether from skin, fat, bone marrow, umbilical cord, or even fetal tissue—is that they can produce growth factors that influence a variety of different cell types, not necessarily of their cell type of origin. They typically take their cues from the cells around them, so if you apply them to the skin, they help generate new skin cells. These new skin cells then can produce more collagen and elastin, and this leads to younger, thicker, more supple skin.

Epidermal growth factor (EGF) is one of the

earliest known growth factors. EGFs directly affect collagen, elastin, and other dermal structures' biosynthesis, though this ability is gradually reduced with age. The topical use of growth factors and cytokines (other signaling proteins that regenerate skin) has been repeatedly shown to be safe and effective when applied to the skin (Fabi and Sundaram, 2014).

The first commercially available product, Tissue Nutrient Serum (SkinMedica) contained human growth factors and cytokines from proteins derived from a culture of fibroblasts of neonatal foreskin (harvested from a single circumcision years before). Clinical data shows that this combination of growth factors and cytokines produce increased collagen and thickening of the skin, decreasing fine lines and improving texture.

Another widely available product, Bio-Restorative skin cream (Neocutis), uses fetal fibroblast cells in culture to produce growth factor and cytokines. While this has created some controversy, it should be noted that the fibroblast cell line came from a fetal skin biopsy following a medically necessary terminated pregnancy. The embryonic environment is a unique one, in which there is rapid stem cell growth and the well-documented phenomenon of scarless healing. Embryos operated on in utero often emerge from the womb with no scars. These fetal fibroblasts are an ideal source of growth factors for skin rejuvenation. Multiple double-blinded studies have shown an increase in epidermal thickness and improvement in appearance of wrinkles.

ReGenica (Allergan), a third product line containing growth factors and cytokines, was developed to simulate the embryonic environment by suspending newborn fibroblast cells on starch beads in low-oxygen conditions. This environment causes them to revert back into stem cells, and start secreting embryonic-like growth factors.

Other products have chosen to remove the human element completely, such as Bioeffect (Bioeffect, Inc.) and Ronald Moy's DNA Renewal Line (Cellular MD). These serums come from a human-like epidermal growth factor that is made from bioengineered barley seeds. Scientists introduced a synthetic DNA into the barley stem cell, which made a protein with the same amino acid sequence as human EGF, so it can easily bind to

EGF receptors on human skin cells. These products have been shown in clinical trials to improve brown spots, skin texture, pore size, and wrinkles.

Other plant-derived human-like growth factors are currently being developed from black cohosh (*Cimicifuga racemosa*) and other plant sources, and it is likely we will see other growth factors bioengineered from plants in the future. There is an argument that bioengineered EGF is purer and more stable in creams than its human counterpart. Plant-generated EGF has a defined concentration of known growth factors. The EGF from human sources uses an undefined extract, a "soup" of many different proteins. This combination of growth factors, cytokines, and other kinds of growth factors influences blood vessel formation, reduces inflammation, and more.

That soup, however, seems to be critical in the creation of human growth factors for skin care products. The fibroblasts from the human donor are grown in a liquid, called a cell culture medium, or broth, which gives the cells the nutrients they need to thrive and produce growth factors and cytokines. That soup may be the essential ingredient in skin care. These human-derived growth factors and their soup may be more active, because they work synergistically with each other.

Nevertheless, some people simply feel uncomfortable with the idea of a human cell line, especially of fetal origin, producing the growth factors that they apply to their skin. The somewhat unpleasant smell of human proteins may also be a deterrent.

Another major hurdle for retailing EGF products is their shelf life. On average, their stability under normal storage conditions is about three months. This can be extended with refrigeration and packaging that protects the product from exposure to air. They are also broken down by acidic environments, so they should not be applied with vitamin C or alpha hydroxy acids.

Safety has also been a concern surrounding growth factors applied to the skin. Since human growth factors have been shown to increase the growth rate of cells, the question has been raised about their effect on malignant cells—namely, if they can promote the growth of cancerous cells in the body. As of now, there is no evidence that products containing growth factors can speed the growth of malignant lesions. The molecules are large, and high quantities cannot be adequately absorbed.

In summary, growth factors from both human and non-human sources have been shown in a significant number of trials to improve the look and texture of skin by stimulating collagen and elastin and increasing blood supply within the skin. They are a beneficial addition to a skin care regimen, and tend to be well tolerated by most people.

Cleansers: The Good, the Bad, and the Irritating

CHAPTER 10

The art of cleansing the skin has come a long way over several thousand years from simply scraping the skin to an exercise in relaxation and a ritual that has both religious and health significance. Early humans cleansed their skin by using pieces of bone or stone to scrape the skin. The earliest recorded evidence of the production of soap-like materials dates back to around 1800 BC in ancient Babylon. Later, the Greeks and Romans used plant materials and animal fat to make soap.

Soaps and cleansers are designed to remove dirt, sebum, and oils from the skin as well as to control bacteria and odor. Most of these do so with the use of surfactants, which are chemical agents that surround dirt and oil, making it easier for water to wash them away.

Until forty years ago, the standard skin cleanser was bar soap. These original bar soaps were very irritating to skin because of their alkaline pH, usually between 9 and 10. They contain sodium salts of fatty acids.

Synthetic detergent bars, also known as **syndet** bars, were developed as an alternative. Syndet bars can be adjusted to the pH of normal skin, between 5 and 6, and produce less irritation and dryness of the skin. Syndet bars contain surfactants such as dioctyl sodium sulfosuccinate and sodium lauryl sulfate. Moisturizing syndet bars have glycerin and other emollients added to help the skin maintain a normal pH level and feel softer.

Deodorant soaps contain the same sodium salts but have an added antibacterial ingredient, such as triclocarban. These soaps often have a pH between 9 and 10 and may cause skin irritation.

Lipid free cleansers are liquid products that clean without soap and water. As the name implies, they contain no fats. They are applied to dry skin, rubbed to produce a lather, and the area is then wiped dry or rinsed off with water. They are suitable for people with dry and/or sensitive skin. These products contain emollients (cetyl alcohol, glycerin) and humectants (propylene glycol) which counter the irritancy or drying potential of the surfactant. They leave behind a thin moisturizing film and can be used effectively to remove makeup in sensitive individuals.

Cleansing creams (cold creams) are applied to the face to both clean and moisturize. They are composed of water, mineral oil, petrolatum, and waxes, and are recommended only for extremely dry skin. They combine the effect of a lipid solvent, such as beeswax, with the detergent action from a substance such as borax.

Liquid body washes are more convenient as well as more hygienic than bar soaps, since multiple individuals do not come into direct contact with the product. They incorporate water and emollients, though their irritancy potential depends mostly on their pH.

Astringents and toners are synonymous terms and refer to a fragranced, diluted alcohol used to remove oil and traces of makeup. They produce a tight or clean feeling that many people find desirable, especially those with acne or oily skin. Many cosmetic cleansing routines recommend using an astringent after washing with a syndet soap. For those who cannot tolerate the dryness and irritation that may come with an alcohol-based toner, alcohol-free toners have been developed. These typically contain witch hazel (derived from a plant that contains anti-inflammatory properties), vinegar, and many other ingredients such as rose water, hyaluronic acid, glycerin, and vitamin C. Most astringents and toners are formulated to restore the normal skin pH of 5 to 6 after cleansing with a more alkaline cleanser.

Exfoliants are products that remove the dead skin cells from the outer layer of the skin. The idea is to remove dead skin cells and uncover new skin that looks brighter, smoother, and more radiant. These products also claim to speed up the natural turnover of skin cells and may stimulate collagen production. Exfoliants may be either mechanical or chemical.

Mechanical exfoliants involve using abrasive devices such as sponges, mitts, dry brushes, or scrubbing granules in a cream or gel base. These granules may be polyethylene beads, aluminum oxide, ground fruit pits, or other synthetic or naturally occurring abrasive materials. Chemical exfoliants contain substances like glycolic acid, salicylic acid, lactic acid, and plant enzymes that promote stratum corneum sloughing.

Exfoliants must be used cautiously. When they are used too vigorously or too frequently, they can cause irritation, especially in sensitive and acne-prone skin.

In summary, skin cleansers have evolved significantly from the simple removal of dirt to the complex, ritualistic elimination of sebum, dead cells, and microorganisms, all while simultaneously maintaining the normal homeostatic environment of the skin. Various formulations of skin cleansers are suitable for different skin types, and it is important to choose a cleanser based on the oiliness, sensitivity, and skin conditions of an individual. There is no one-size-fits-all cleanser for the skin.

Hair Products: Shining, Gleaming, Streaming

CHAPTER 11

Throughout history, hair has played a significant role in our society. It is associated with youthfulness and beauty in women and virility and masculinity in men. It is no surprise that there are thousands of products available to consumers to cleanse, style, color, curl, straighten, and grow hair.

To understand hair products, it is important to understand hair. Hair is not as simple as it may seem; it is a complex structure that varies from one race to another and from one individual to another.

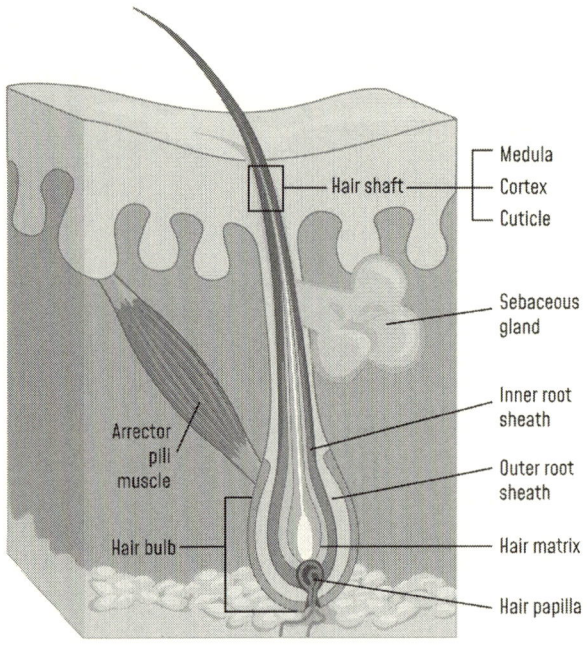

Hair grows from a pocket in the skin called the hair follicle, or the pore. There are approximately 100,000 hair follicles on the average head, and we typically lose about 100 to 200 hairs daily. Hair grows about one-eighth of an inch per day, and it grows in repeated five to seven year cycles. Hair color and baldness in both men and women are both genetically determined.

Hair is made up of three structures: the cuticle, the cortex, and the medulla. The cuticle is the outside of the hair shaft, and it is the part that everyone sees. It is made of five to ten overlapping layers of protein (keratin), like shingles on a roof. The cuticle is thickest in Asian hair, slightly less in Caucasian hair, and even less in African hair. The thinner cuticle in African hair makes it more prone to breakage. The cuticle protects the cortex underneath, which is the middle section of the hair shaft. The cortex contains long bundles of proteins that give hair its strength and keep it from breaking. At the very center of the hair is the medulla, which is an empty zone that helps insulate the hair. Not all hair contains a medulla; it is found in coarser hair like grey hair, thick hair, and beard hair, and is absent in the fine hair of children. The medulla provides an area of weakness in the hair, and may contribute to splitting of hairs. Each hair is covered by a natural lipid layer, sebum, which helps the hair fiber resist water and chemical treatments.

Afro-ethnic hair is distinct in that the diameter varies at several points along the fiber (the diameter at the twisting points is smaller than at other areas), has less water content, has a more oval cross-section than Caucasian hair, and has a thinner cuticle. This makes the hair more susceptible to breakage and more difficult to comb without provoking frizz.

Hair damage can result when the natural lipid layer of the hair is removed, causing the hair to absorb water. Wet, virgin hair can be stretched by 30 percent of its original length without damage; however, irreversible changes occur when hair is stretched between 30 percent and 70 percent. Stretching to 80 percent causes fracture of the hair. Excessive or repeated chemical treatment, grooming habits (such as backcombing), and environmental exposure produce changes in hair texture, and ultimately cause hair breakage. These changes can be seen microscopically as weathering of the hair shaft, and contribute to tangling and frizzing. When hair is extremely weathered and chemically treated, there may be scaling of the cuticle layers, removal of the lipid layer, and cuticle cracking. Once the cortex is exposed from the loss of the protective cuticle layer, the hair is prone to fracture, which we see as splitting and breaking of the hair fiber.

Shampoos were initially designed to remove dirt and oil from the hair and scalp. While this may sound like a simple task, most consumers want a shampoo that beautifies as well. Hair that has had all the sebum removed is dull in appearance, coarse to the touch, and is difficult to manage and style.

Shampoos function by employing detergents, also known as surfactants, that contain molecules with both lipophilic (oil-loving) and hydrophilic (water-loving) portions. The oil-loving end attaches to the grease and dirt in your hair and the water-loving end allows the water in the shower to rinse away the oil with the shampoo. The most common detergents in shampoos are fatty alcohol sulfates, and have names like sodium lauryl sulfate, sodium laureth sulfate, and ammonium laureth sulfate. Sulfates are very effective in removing grease and dirt, and are easy to rinse out. They are good at cleansing, but can be hard on the hair. Many people have a negative view of sulfates in shampoo, because they can strip away too much moisture, leaving the hair dry and unmanageable, so sulfate-free shampoos have been created. There is no risk to a person's health from using shampoo containing sulfates, although sulfate-free shampoos often leave the hair feeling not as clean. However, they can be good choices for chemically treated or very dry hair.

Foaming agents in shampoos introduce gas bubbles into the water, and many consumers believe that shampoos that generate copious foam are better cleansers. This is not true. Foam is not necessary for adequate cleansing.

Conditioning shampoos are simply shampoos with the addition of a conditioner. It is questionable whether a product can clean and condition at the same time. Conditioning shampoos may actually be self-defeating, since the shampoo is intended to remove sebum, the body's natural conditioner, and replace it with a synthetic conditioner at the same time. As a result, conditioning shampoos typically neither clean nor condition well.

Another advertising claim made by some manufacturers is that their formulation is "pH balanced." Most shampoos, like skin cleansers, are alkaline, which can swell the hair shaft and make it more susceptible to damage. This is usually not a problem for people with healthy hair with intact cuticles. However, if the hair is damaged or chemically treated, it may be better to use a shampoo with an acid added to bring the pH closer to hair's natural pH of 4 to 5.

Hair conditioners are used to decrease friction, detangle the hair, minimize frizz and make combing wet hair easier. The need for conditioners arose following the development of shampoos with extremely good cleansing action. The newer shampoos so thoroughly removed sebum from the hair shaft that the hair became dull, unmanageable, and coarse to the touch.

Conditioners neutralize the negative electrical charge of the hair fiber by adding positive charges and also by lubricating the cuticle. Conditioners smooth the cuticle scales down to the hair shaft, reducing friction when the wet hair is combed. Deep conditioners are typically creamier but are otherwise no different from instant conditioners, despite advertisers' claims that they penetrate more deeply and condition better. Most of the effect of a conditioner is accomplished right after it is spread through the hair, and there is little benefit to leaving it on longer.

Hair straighteners, often called chemical relaxers, have a permanent straightening effect on the hair, and the process is similar to permanent waving or curling. The treatment needs to be repeated every twelve weeks or so to straighten the new hair growth. Most permanent straighteners are alkaline, and contain sodium hydroxide, lithium hydroxide, or calcium hydroxide. The high pH of the product swells the hair and opens up the cuticle scales, allowing the product to penetrate into the cortex, where it reacts with the keratin, breaking and rearranging the disulfide bridges. The hair is then mechanically straightened with a comb to restructure the position of the disulfide bonds. If these chemicals are applied with poor technique, they can cause scalp burns and hair breakage.

Brazilian keratin treatments (the Brazilian blowout) are temporary straightening and smoothing salon treatments to make hair look smoother, fuller, and glossier. The Brazilian keratin treatment uses a liquid keratin to coat each strand of hair. In order to bond the keratin to the hair shaft, other chemicals, such as formaldehyde, are needed. The Brazilian blowout solutions have been shown to contain up to 12 percent formaldehyde. The

FDA classified formaldehyde as a cancer-causing chemical in 1987. It has been linked to leukemia and some cancers in the nose. It has also been associated with childhood leukemias in mothers exposed to formaldehyde during pregnancy.

There are newer Brazilian keratin treatments that claim to be formaldehyde free, but some of these products contain formaldehyde-releasers, so they may carry the same risk. Pregnant women should avoid these products, and salon operatives and customers should use protective measures, such as mask and gloves.

Hair coloring agents are a common hair cosmetic used by both men and women. At least 40 percent of women use some type of coloring agent. There are many types of hair dyes classified according to how deeply they penetrate the hair shaft. For purposes of this discussion, we will look at the two most commonly used types of hair dye: permanent and semi-permanent.

The main difference between the dyes is their capacity to either reach the cortex of the hair shaft and remain there permanently, or to simply stay on the surface of the cuticle and be washed out after about ten to fifteen shampoos; the latter are the so-called semi-permanent dyes.

Permanent hair colors are the most commonly used hair colors because of their longevity. The pigmentation is permanent, and the original hair color that shows up ten to fifteen days after the application of the dye is not due to removal of the dye by shampoo, but is due to new hair growth. Permanent dyes have an alkaline pH to open the scales of the cuticle and allow the pigment to penetrate the cortex. Most contain ammonia and hydrogen peroxide. These dyes cause weakening of the hair shaft, making it prone to breaking and splitting.

Semi-permanent dyes are gentler on the hair than the permanent colors. They are not as effective in coloring grey or white hair and cannot lighten the shade of the hair, since they only coat the cuticle with pigment and do not reach the cortex. They wash out after ten to fifteen shampoos or less, but cause much less damage to the hair.

Techniques for damaged hair are as important as products designed to reverse damage, but it is amazing how much money consumers will spend on damaging their hair through chemical processing and then subsequently on suboptimal attempts to repair the damage (Draelos, 1990).

The most important rule for chemically damaged hair is to subject it to as little physical stress as possible. Styling, including combing and brushing, should be kept to a minimum. Hair should be washed gently and a conditioner applied before combing; wet hair should be combed with the utmost care. Heat styling (hair dryers and hot rollers) should be avoided or used for as short a period as possible. Hair dryers should be held at least twelve inches away from the hair surface, and should be kept in continual motion during the drying process. Tight hair clasps and rubber bands pulling on the hair should be avoided or used only occasionally.

In summary, humans will never stop using hair cosmetics and mechanically treating their hair. The use of gentler, pH balanced products and minimizing physical stress to the hair can help reverse a portion of that damage, but decreasing shampooing and chemical treatments will make the biggest difference.

Nail Products: Tools, Not Jewels

Humans have nails to protect the sensitive tips of the fingers and toes. Nails also increase the dexterity of hands, allowing us to pick up small objects. Without them, we would have a hard time scratching an itch or untying a knot.

Nails grow out of the deep folds in the skin of the fingers and toes. Nails are formed in the matrix, which is an area beneath the fold at the base of the nail. As the nail cells accumulate, the nail pushes forward and grows. Fingernails grow faster than toenails. Like hair, nails grow faster in the summer than in the winter. A nail that has torn off or been surgically removed will grow back as long as the matrix is not severely damaged.

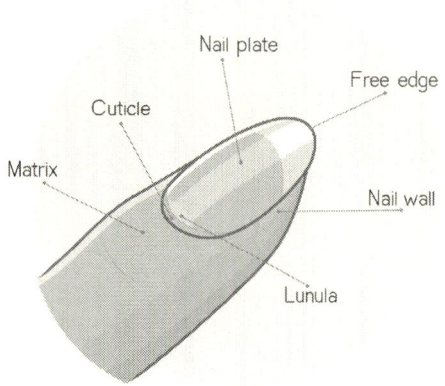

Nail art and adornment dates back to around 3000 BC in China, where evidence of long, manicured nails has been found in early Chinese art. In some of this art, nails are depicted as extremely long, indicating the relative priority of form over function. Nail art and adornment have expanded exponentially in the last few years. Each month, Google logs over three million searches for "nail art."

The most common nail products are nail enamels (polish), nail hardeners, nail enamel removers, cuticle removers, and artificial nails.

Nail enamels contain various colored pigments suspended in a film former. The most common film former is nitrocellulose, a highly flammable substance that creates a film that adheres to the nail. This creates a coating on the nail that provides hardness and resistance to abrasion. Polishes also often contain toluene sulfonamide formaldehyde to increase flexibility, but this compound is highly allergenic and many polishes, especially those labelled hypoallergenic, have removed the compound.

One problem associated with nail enamels is a yellow discoloration of the nail after the enamel is removed, especially with deeper and darker pigments. This is often mistaken for a fungal infection, but it is simply staining of the nail and will usually disappear after a few weeks without polish.

Nail hardeners, as their name implies, are designed to harden or strengthen the nail, and allow the nail to reach a longer length before breakage occurs. Originally, nail hardeners contained formaldehyde (often listed as formalin or methylene glycol), but that proved to be a common cause of allergic reactions, so it is no longer used in nail hardener preparations. Nylon, acrylics, and polyamide resins are now used instead.

Nail enamel removers are used to remove enamel from the nail. Liquid removers are most popular, and usually contain acetone, alcohol, and ethyl acetate. These can cause irritation of the skin around the nail, as well as dehydration and brittleness of the nail itself. Conditioning nail enamel removers are an attempt to combat this irritation, and contain fatty acids such as cetyl alcohol, lanolin, and oils. Scents and colors may also be added for cosmetic appeal.

Cuticle removers dissolve excess tissue around and on the nail. However, cuticles exist for a very important reason. They provide a watertight protection for the nail matrix, which is that very critical area where the nail is formed, and where damage can result in a permanently abnormal or misshapen nail. Since visible cuticle is not considered aesthetically pleasing, thorough removal of any noticeable cuticle is part of the complete manicure or pedicure. Cuticle removers contain two to five percent sodium or potassium hydroxide, a powerful skin irritant—remember, their goal is to dissolve skin cells! When this watertight boundary is removed, bacteria and yeast can invade the space around the nail, causing inflammation or infection, known as a paronychia. When this becomes chronic, it can result in an abnormal or deformed nail. Most dermatologists do not advocate removing the cuticle.

Artificial nails are divided into sculptured nails, press-on nails, and nail wrapping.

Sculptured nails are the most common artificial nail preparations. These consist of acrylic polymers in a liquid preparation, which is applied to the entire nail and can be formed into whatever shape or length is desired. They are then sanded and enamel may be applied. The sculptured nail loosens and begins to grow out after two to three weeks, and new acrylic must be applied around the edges (so-called "filling").

In the early 1970s, the FDA received a number of complaints of injury associated with the use of artificial nails containing methyl methacrylate monomer. Among these injuries were reports of fingernail damage and deformity, as well as contact dermatitis. Unlike methyl methacrylate monomer, ethyl methacrylate polymers were not associated with these injuries. Based on these reports, the FDA removed products from the market that contained methyl methacrylate monomer.

Unfortunately, there are still many problems with sculptured nails. Many states do not require licensing of operators, so there is no regulation of operator training, application technique, and hygiene. Poorly trained operators may allow the liquid acrylic to seep into the matrix, causing permanent nail damage. Failure to properly clean and sterilize equipment can result in bacterial and fungal infections around the nail.

Even with proper application, use of sculptured nails causes the natural nail to become yellowed, dry, and thin. The nails are more prone to becoming separated from the fingertip skin. Therefore, it is not advisable to wear sculptured nails for more than three months at a time. One month should be allowed between applications to allow the nail to grow naturally and regain strength.

Press-on nails are pre-formed plastic nails that come in a variety of sizes and shapes. They are glued onto the natural nail with an acrylic-based cement, which is a potential source of an allergic reaction. The major danger of these nails is damage to the nail and lifting of the nail when they are left in place for prolonged periods.

Nail wrapping is the technique of applying tissue paper, silk, or linen cloth to the nail to provide strength. After placement of the mesh on the nail, multiple layers of liquid acrylic are applied to seal the cloth. Again, the major drawbacks are damage to the nail when the nail wrap is left on for a long time as well as allergic reactions to the acrylic.

In summary, many of the techniques used to strengthen and beautify the nails can lead to damage, infection, and allergic reaction. The best policy is to use nail cosmetic products temporarily (no more than three months at a time), and then allow the nail to grow naturally for at least one month.

Acne Products: I'm Too Old For This!

CHAPTER 13

Yes, adults get acne. Acne is frustrating no matter when it occurs, but it can be particularly embarrassing for adults. Adult acne can continue well into your thirties, forties, and even fifties. It is even possible to develop acne for the first time as an adult.

Acne pimples occur when the pores are clogged with a combination of dead skin cells, oil (sebum), and bacteria. Pores, which are the openings that surround each hair follicle, are an important part of the skin because they also house the sebaceous glands. These glands secrete sebum (oil) through the pore opening, which helps keep your skin soft and protected. When the pore is clogged by dirt, dead skin cells, oil, and possibly bacteria, inflammation occurs and the result is a pimple.

Women tend to get adult acne more often than men. When acne occurs as an adult, it is likely due to one or more of the following reasons:

Fluctuating hormone levels. Hormonal factors related to estrogen and progesterone are probably the most important cause of adult acne in women. Fluctuations in hormones occur around the time of the menstrual period, during or after pregnancy, during perimenopause and menopause, and after starting or stopping birth control pills. Androgens (male hormones) like testosterone can increase sebum production and can play a role in hormonal acne in people of both genders.

Stress. Researchers have found a relationship between stress and acne flare-ups. Stress causes the adrenal gland to release cortisol (the body's natural cortisone) as well as androgens (male hormones). Chronic stress can produce a favorable environment for inflammatory acne to develop within the hair follicle.

Skin and hair products. If you have adult acne, you should read the labels on your skin care and hair care products. You should be using only products that are labeled oil-free, non-comedogenic, or non-acnegenic. All of your products, including cleanser, moisturizer, sunscreen, and foundation should contain these terms. These products are less likely to clog pores and cause acne. However, a good rule of thumb is to minimize the number of products you apply to your skin. Sunscreen (oil-free and non-acnegenic) is essential to use daily, but moisturizers and other cosmetics should be used sparingly.

An underlying medical condition. In a small percentage of patients, acne can be caused by an undiagnosed medical condition. In women, a disorder called polycystic ovary syndrome (PCOS) often underlies chronic or difficult to control acne. Symptoms also include menstrual irregularity, excess hair growth, and obesity. A careful medical history review and physical exam, including some possible laboratory tests, can better identify underlying medical causes of acne.

Family history. Findings from research studies suggest that some people may have a genetic predisposition for acne. If a close relative, such as a parent, brother, or sister has acne, your acne may be genetically predisposed. The good news is that does not mean it cannot be treated.

Medications. Some medications have the side effect of either causing acne or making it worse.

Common medications include steroids (including oral, cream, and inhaled forms), birth control pills, lithium, and testosterone, to name a few. Your doctor should be able to determine if a medication is contributing to your acne, and, if so, either replace it with a different drug or continue it and treat the acne.

Diet. The relationship between diet and acne is not clear and is currently under debate. A large review of the literature in 2004 (Wolf et al, 2004) concluded that there was no convincing evidence of the effects of diet on acne. However, another review in that same year linked acne to milk consumption (Adebamowo et al, 2005) The investigators in that study raised the point that the majority of milk and dairy products consumed in the United States come from pregnant cows. Could these products contribute to acne because they expose us to the hormones the cows produce when they are pregnant? Investigations of the effect of dairy products on acne are ongoing.

Some recent studies have suggested that a high glycemic index diet may increase the severity of acne. The American Academy of Dermatology has stated that (a) no specific dietary changes are recommended in the treatment of acne, (b) emerging data suggests that high glycemic index diets may be associated with acne, and (c) limited evidence suggests that some dairy products, particularly skim milk, may influence acne.

The rule of thumb is to pay attention to your skin, and if you feel that avoiding certain foods improves your acne, it is probably wise to avoid those foods.

Is Effective Treatment for Adult Acne Available?

The simple answer is yes. Treatments may include a combination of topical products, cleansers, exfoliants, and oral medications. Some of these are available over the counter, and some require a physician's prescription. Remember, acne is a medical condition—do not hesitate to seek medical attention just as you would for any health condition if your acne does not respond to over-the-counter medications. With patience, nearly every case of acne can be treated and controlled.

Topical Treatments

There are numerous products containing science-backed ingredients available over the counter. It is important to realize that not every product works the same for everyone, and many of these products need to be used consistently for a few weeks before their effects are noticeable. Treating acne with acne products takes time and patience. It may take two or three months of daily use of an acne product to see results. Acne may look worse before it gets better.

Benzoyl peroxide is an ingredient that has been around for years and is very effective at treating acne. Benzoyl peroxide works to treat and prevent acne by killing bacteria that cause acne; it also helps pores shed dead skin cells and excess sebum. Available in over-the-counter gels, cleansers, and spot treatments, this ingredient also comes in different concentrations ranging from 2.5 percent to 10 percent

While benzoyl peroxides are considered safe for most people, they also have some potential side effects. Because they cause dead skin cells to peel and reduce sebum, they can cause dryness, as well as redness and excessive peeling. They also have the potential for allergic reactions in the skin, which results in itching, redness, and a rash. Be careful when applying benzoyl peroxide as it can bleach hair and clothing.

Salicylic acid helps pores from becoming plugged by dissolving the bonds between dead skin cells. Salicylic acid is particularly helpful when treating acne because it is oil soluble, which allows it to penetrate deeper into the hair follicle where the oil-producing sebaceous glands reside. Salicylic acid products are available in strengths ranging from 0.5 percent to 5 percent.

Alpha hydroxy acids are a group of natural acids that help to remove dead skin cells and stimulate the growth of new, smoother skin (discussed in Chapter 5). They are water-soluble, so they do not have the benefit of being attracted to the oily pore; they can, however, improve the appearance of the skin and give the impression of smaller pores. They come in multiple strengths, with the higher concentrations being more powerful but also more sensitizing.

Sulfur removes dead skin cells that clog pores and helps remove excess oil. It is often combined with other ingredients, such as salicylic acid, benzoyl peroxide, or resorcinol. Products containing sulfur may cause dry skin, and some products have an unpleasant odor.

Azelaic acid works by killing the bacteria in pores that cause acne and by decreasing the production of keratin, produced by dead skin cells. Azelaic acid is also an effective treatment for rosacea, causing decreased swelling and redness of the skin.

Retinoids are vitamin A derivatives and include tretinoin, retinol, retinaldehyde, tazarotene, and adapalene. All are available over the counter, except tretinoin and tazarotene. Topical retinoids are some of the most effective treatments for acne, and have beneficial anti-aging ingredients (discussed in Chapter 6).

Retinoids work by promoting the turnover and exfoliation of dead skin cells as well as boosting the production of new skin cells. These new skin cells then push dead cells and excess oil out of blocked pores. In addition, retinoids have anti-inflammatory properties.

While retinoids are safe for most people, they

can have some side effects. The most common side effects are mild skin irritation, such as itching, peeling, flaking, and burning. They can also cause a worsening of acne at the beginning of treatment. These problems generally resolve within a few weeks of starting therapy.

The most important side effect of retinoids is an increased sensitivity to sunlight, which can lead to severe sunburn. It is vital when using a retinoid to be vigilant about using sunscreen and to stay out of direct sunlight as much as possible. Like the other side effects of retinoids, this also tends to diminish with time.

Oral Medications

Depending on the root cause and severity of your acne, over-the-counter topical products may not be successful, and it may be necessary to consult a dermatologist who may recommend an oral medication.

Antibiotics. For moderate to severe acne, you may need oral antibiotics to reduce bacteria in the hair follicle and treat inflammatory acne lesions. Common choices are the tetracyclines (minocycline, doxycycline) or a macrolide (erythromycin, azithromycin).

Oral antibiotics should be used for the shortest time possible to minimize drug resistance. They are frequently combined with topical medications.

Oral contraceptives. The FDA has approved a number of combined oral contraceptives for acne therapy in women who also wish to use them for birth control. These products combine progestin and estrogen.

You may not see the benefit of this treatment for a few months, so it is usually combined with other acne medications, at least in the beginning.

Anti-androgen agents. Spironolactone can be used in women and post-adolescent girls if oral antibiotics are not helping. It works by blocking the effect of androgen (male) hormones on the oil-producing glands.

Isotretinoin is an oral derivative of vitamin A. It is prescribed for moderate to severe acne that has not responded to other treatments.

Isotretinoin has potential serious side effects, and requires regular monitoring by a physician and participation in an FDA-approved risk management program.

In summary, acne is seen not only in children and teenagers but in adults through their sixth decade. Depending on the severity and cause, abundant effective treatments are available over the counter, and when that is not effective, prescription medications may be necessary. Most acne can be treated and controlled at any age.

Preservatives: To Preserve or Not to Preserve

CHAPTER 14

Everyone knows that food can go bad. Leave a loaf of bread on the counter for too long and it will sprout fuzzy green or white mold. However, food is not the only thing with a shelf life. Skin care products and cosmetics have shelf lives too, which is why they usually contain preservatives.

The FDA defines a preservative as a "substance of natural or synthetic origin intended to inhibit the development of microorganisms. This inhibition should be effective over a broad activity spectrum and should have a duration longer than the cosmetic product itself."

Have there been any major health problems from contamination in skin care products? Absolutely. The *New York Times* reported that bacteria-contaminated facial lotions caused a small outbreak of blindness in the 1950s, which then led to the use of parabens in cosmetics. Through the years, there have been a number of recalls of cosmetic products due to contamination with bacteria and mold.

Preservatives are not the enemy. Unpreserved products can lose potency or become contaminated with harmful microbial agents. Products can become contaminated while they are being used, during the manufacturing process, or from exposure to light and air. Many disease-causing bacteria, fungi, and yeasts have been cultured from skin care products.

The design of a product—for example, whether it is in a sealed or an open container—can play a role in potential contamination. Products that come with applicators, such as mascara wands, are exposed to bacteria and fungi every time they are used. As the FDA states on its website, products can become contaminated through finger contact, especially open-top jars.

Water is an ideal growth medium for microorganisms. Since most products contain some percentage of water, they provide favorable environments for microbial growth. In general, the lower the ratio of water to oil in a product, the less favorable the environment is for growth of microorganisms.

The pH, or acidity, of a product also influences its potential for contamination. The optimal pH for microbial growth in cosmetic products is between 5 and 8, meaning that any pH outside this range makes a less favorable environment for the growth of microorganisms. A product containing an acid, such as an alpha hydroxy acid (with a pH of 3 to 4), makes contamination much less likely.

Preservatives used in skin care products can be divided into three categories: natural, synthetic, and chemical.

Natural preservatives include vitamins C and E, honey, thyme and rosemary extract, and tea tree oil. While the concept of natural preservatives may sound appealing to some, these ingredients do not provide effective protection against bacteria and other microbes from contaminating products when used alone.

Synthetic preservatives include food grade sodium benzoate and derivatives of alcohol, such as ethanol and benzyl alcohol, and propylene glycol. These ingredients have proven safety profiles.

Chemical preservatives include parabens, formaldehyde, and diazolidinyl urea. This category of preservatives has been flagged by some consumer watchdog associations as potentially unsafe. These products are currently being further investigated for safety.

Conclusion

CHAPTER 15

The skin care market can seem formidable to even the most discerning consumer. With a market share well in the billions and little oversight by an overworked FDA, the average person must determine which products actually are effective and are worth the money. With over 80 percent of product claims being either misleading or untruthful, the burden is on the consumer to read the label and evaluate the ingredients.

I have attempted to provide information about ingredients which are backed by scientific data, meaning clinical studies published in medical journals. I have avoided giving brand names except in a few instances, so it is important for the serious consumer to become fluent in the language of product ingredients. Don't be scared by long chemical names—they can usually be broken down into understandable components.

The good news is that there are products that

work—and many are available at affordable prices. One fact has become clear to me in my research—price and effectiveness are very often unrelated. Department stores, drug stores and online markets all provide products with proven effectiveness, often at very different price points.

So—take product claims with a grain of salt—and read the ingredients. And remember—looking and feeling good at ANY age is antiaging!

REFERENCES

1. Fowler, Jie G, et al. Deception in cosmetics advertising: Examining cosmetics advertising claims in fashion magazine ads. *Journal of Global Fashion Marketing*, 2015; 6 (3): 194 DOI: 10.1080/20932685.2015.1032319.
2. Wood, L. Global Cosmetics Market—By Product Type, Ingredient, Geography, and Vendors—Market Size, Demand Forecasts, Industry Trends and Updates, Supplier Market Shares 2014–2020. URL: Research and Markets. Available online: https://www.researchandmarkets.com/research/f2lvdg/global_cosmetics.
3. Gilchrest, B. Skin Aging and Photoaging: An Overview. *J. Amer Assn of Dermatol*. 1989: 3, 310-613.
4. Gilchrest, B. A Review of Skin Ageing and its Medical Therapy. *Brit Assn of Dermatol*. 1996: 135, 867-875.

5. Drake, L. et al. Guidelines of care for photoaging/photodamage. *J Amer Acad Dermatol.* 1996:35, 462-465.
6. Cerimele, D. et al. Physiological changes in ageing skin. 1970: *Br J Dermatol.* 35 (suppl), 13-20.
7. Guy GP, et al. Prevalence and costs of skin cancer treatment in the US, 2002–2006 and 2007–2011. *Am J Prev Med.* 2015;48:183–7.
8. Suh S. et al The banned sunscreen ingredients and their impact on human health: A systematic review. *Int. J. Dermatol.* 2020;59:1033–1042.
9. Schneider, S. and Lim, H. Review of environmental effects of oxybenzone and other sunscreen active ingredients. *J Amer Acad Dermatol.* 2018:80:266-271.
10. Wang, Steven Q., Mark E. Burnett, and Henry W. Lim. "Safety of Oxybenzone: Putting Numbers Into Perspective." *Archives of Dermatology* 2011;14 (7): 865-866.
11. Neale, RE et al. The effect of sunscreen on vitamin D: a review. *Br J Dermatol .* 2019; 181:907.
12. Watts. CG et al. Sunscreen use and melanoma risk among young Australian adults. *JAMA Dermatol* 2018; 154: 1001.

13. Maier, T and Korting, HC. Sunscreens—Which and What For? *Skin Pharmacol Physiol.* 2005: 18, 253-262.
14. Lin, J. The Science of Sunscreen. Harvard Health Publishing, www.health.harvard.edu, 4/5/21.
15. Draelos, Z. (1990) Cosmetics in Dermatology. Churchill Livingstone.
16. Sethi, A. et al. Moisturizers: The Slippery Road. *Indian J Dermatol. 2016: 61, 279-287.*
17. Ditre, SM et al. Effects of alpha hydroxy acids on photoaged skin: A pilot clinical, histologic, and ultrastructural study. *J Am Acad Dermatol.* 1996: 35, 187-195.
18. Martin, K. and Glaser, D. Cosmeceuticals: The New Medicine of Beauty. *Missouri Medicine.* 2011: 108, 60-63.
19. Weiss, J. et al. Topical Tretinoin improves photoaged skin. *JAMA.* 1988: 259, 527-532.
20. Kang, S and Voorhees, J. Photoaging therapy with topical tretinoin: an evidence-based analysis. *J Am Acad Dermatol.* 1998: 39, #55-S61.
21. Farris, P. et al. The mechanism of action of topical retinoids for the treatment of

nonmalignant photodamage. *Cos Dermatol.* 2010: 23, 19-24.
22. Mukherjee, S. et al. Retinoids in the treatment of skin aging. *Clin Interv Aging.* 2006: 1 (4), 1-35.
23. Bhawan, J. et al. Effects of tretinoin on photodamaged skin: a histologic study. *Arch Dermatol.* 1991: 127, 666-72.
24. Kang et al. Application of retinol to human skin in vivo induces epidermal hyperplasia and cellular retinoid binding proteins characteristic of retinoic acid but without measurable retinoic acid levels or irritation. *J Invest Dermatol.* 1995: 105, 549-56.
25. Kang et al. A multicenter, randomized, double-blind trial of tazarotene 0.1 percent cream in the treatment of photodamage. *J Am Acad Dermatol.* 2005: 52, 268-74.
26. Schagen, S. Topical peptide treatments with effective anti-aging results. *Cosmetics.* 2017: 4(2):16.
27. Addor, F. Antioxidants in Dermatology. *An Bras Dermatol.* 2017: 92(3), 356-362.
28. Fabi, S. and Sundaram, H. The potential of topical and injectable growth factors and

cytokines for skin rejuvenation. *Facial Plast Surg.* 2014: 30, 157-71.
29. Aldag, C. et al. Skin rejuvenation using cosmetic products containing growth factor, cytokines, and matrikines: a review of the literature. *Clin Cosmet Investig Dermatol.* 2016: 9, 411-419.
30. Eskins, O. and Amin, S. Challenges and effective routes for formulating and delivery of epidermal growth factors in skin care. *Int J Cosmet Sci.* 2020: 43, 123-130.
31. Draelos, Z. (1990). Cosmetics and Cosmeceuticals. In: Bolognia, J et al, editors. *Dermatology.* 2nd ed. Philadelphia: Mosby Elsevier; 2008, 2301-2.
32. Mukhopadhyay, P. Cleansers and their role in various dermatological disorders. *Indian J Dermatol.* 2011:56,2-6.
33. Walters, R. et al. Cleansing formulations that respect skin barrier integrity. *Dermatol Res Pract.* 2012: 495917. doi:10.1155/2012/495917.
34. Reis Gavazzoni Dias, MF. Hair cosmetics: and overview. *Int J Trichology.* 2015 Jan-Mar; 7 (1): 2-15.

35. Gubitosa, J et al. Hair care cosmetics: from traditional shampoo to solid clay and herbal shampoo, a review. *Cosmetics.* 2019: 1-23.
36. Scher, R. Cosmetic and ancillary preparations for the care of nails. *J Amer Acad Dermatol.* 1982 Apr; 6: 23-530.
37. Vlahovic, T. A closer look at cosmetic solution for nails. *Podiatry Today.* 2014.
38. Wolf, R. et al. Acne and diet. *Clin Dermatol.* 2004; 22: 387-393.
39. Adebamowo, CA et al. High school dietary dairy intake and teenage acne. *J Acad Dermatol. 2005;* 52: 207-214.
40. Zaenglein, A. et al. Guidelines of care for the management of acne vulgaris. *J Acad Dermatol.* 2016; 74.
41. Cerman, AA et al. Dietary glycemic factors, insulin resistance, and adiponectin levels in acne vulgaris. *J Acad Dermatol.* 2016; 75: 155-162.
42. Halla, N. et al. Cosmetics preservation: a review on present strategies. *Molecules.* 2018 Jul; 23 (7), 1571.
43. www.FDA.gov/cosmetics/cosmetic-ingredients/parabens-cosmetics.

Made in the USA
Coppell, TX
11 May 2023